Expanded Access to Investigational Drugs for Treatment Use — Questions and Answers

Guidance for Industry

Additional copies are available from:

Office of Communications, Division of Drug Information
Center for Drug Evaluation and Research
Food and Drug Administration
10001 New Hampshire Ave., Hillandale Bldg., 4th Floor
Silver Spring, MD 20993-0002
Phone: 855-543-3784 or 301-796-3400; Fax: 301-431-6353
Email: druginfo@fda.hhs.gov
http://www.fda.gov/Drugs/GuidanceComplianceRegulatoryInformation/Guidances/default.htm

and/or

Office of Communication, Outreach and Development
Center for Biologics Evaluation and Research
Food and Drug Administration
10903 New Hampshire Ave., Bldg. 71, Room 3128
Silver Spring, MD 20993-0002
Phone: 800-835-4709 or 240-402-8010
Email: ocod@fda.hhs.gov
http://www.fda.gov/BiologicsBloodVaccines/GuidanceComplianceRegulatoryInformation/Guidances/default.htm

Food and Drug Administration
Center for Drug Evaluation and Research (CDER)
Center for Biologics Evaluation and Research (CBER)

June 2016
Procedural

Contains Nonbinding Recommendations

TABLE OF CONTENTS

Expanded Access to Investigational Drugs for Treatment Use — Questions and Answers Guidance for Industry[1]

> This guidance represents the current thinking of the Food and Drug Administration (FDA or Agency) on this topic. It does not establish any rights for any person and is not binding on FDA or the public. You can use an alternative approach if it satisfies the requirements of the applicable statutes and regulations. To discuss an alternative approach, contact the FDA office responsible for this guidance as listed on the title page.

I. INTRODUCTION

This guidance provides information for industry, researchers, physicians, institutional review boards (IRBs), and patients about the implementation of FDA's regulations on expanded access to investigational drugs[2] for treatment use under an investigational new drug application (IND) (21 CFR part 312, subpart I), which went into effect on October 13, 2009.[3] Since 2009, FDA has received a number of questions concerning implementation of the regulations. As a result, FDA is providing guidance in a question and answer format, addressing the most frequently asked questions. In a separate guidance,[4] FDA provides answers to questions concerning the implementation of the regulation on charging for investigational drugs under an IND (21 CFR 312.8).[5] Also in a separate guidance, FDA describes Form FDA 3926 (Individual Patient Expanded Access—Investigational New Drug Application (IND)) and the process for submitting expanded access requests for individual patient INDs.[6]

---

[1] This guidance has been prepared by the Office of Medical Policy in the Center for Drug Evaluation and Research in cooperation with the Center for Biologics Evaluation and Research at the Food and Drug Administration.

[2] For the purposes of this guidance, the terms *investigational new drug, investigational drug, drug*, and *drug product* refer to both human drugs and biological drug products regulated by the Center for Drug Evaluation and Research or the Center for Biologics Evaluation and Research.

[3] *Federal Register* of August 13, 2009 (74 FR 40900).

[4] See the guidance for industry *Charging for Investigational Drugs under an IND—Questions and Answers* for the Agency's current thinking on this topic. We update guidance documents periodically. To make sure you have the most recent version of a guidance, check the FDA guidance Web page at http://www.fda.gov/RegulatoryInformation/Guidances/.

[5] See also 74 FR 40872, August 13, 2009.

[6] See the guidance for industry *Individual Patient Expanded Access Applications: Form FDA 3926*.

In general, FDA's guidance documents do not establish legally enforceable responsibilities. Instead, guidances describe the Agency's current thinking on a topic and should be viewed only as recommendations, unless specific regulatory or statutory requirements are cited. The use of the word *should* in Agency guidances means that something is suggested or recommended, but not required.

II.   BACKGROUND

Expanded access refers to the use of an investigational drug when the primary purpose is to diagnose, monitor, or treat a patient rather than to obtain the kind of information about the drug that is generally derived from clinical trials. FDA has a long history of facilitating expanded access to investigational drugs for treatment use for patients with serious or immediately life-threatening diseases or conditions[7] who lack therapeutic alternatives. FDA revised its IND regulations in 2009[8] by removing the existing regulations on treatment use and creating subpart I of part 312 to consolidate and expand the various provisions regarding expanded access to treatment use of investigational drugs.

Under FDA's current regulations, there are three categories of expanded access:

- Expanded access for individual patients, including for emergency use (21 CFR 312.310)

- Expanded access for intermediate-size patient populations (generally smaller than those typical of a treatment IND or treatment protocol — a treatment protocol is submitted as a protocol to an existing IND by the sponsor of the existing IND)[9] (21 CFR 312.315)

- Expanded access for widespread treatment use through a treatment IND or treatment protocol (designed for use in larger patient populations) (21 CFR 312.320)

The revised regulations were, among other things, intended to increase awareness and knowledge about expanded access and the procedures for obtaining investigational drugs for treatment use for patients with serious or immediately life-threatening diseases or conditions who lack therapeutic alternatives. The regulations were also intended to facilitate the availability, when

---

[7] For the purpose of expanded access to investigational drugs for treatment use, immediately life-threatening disease or condition means a stage of disease in which there is reasonable likelihood that death will occur within a matter of months or in which premature death is likely without early treatment. Serious disease or condition means a disease or condition associated with morbidity that has substantial impact on day-to-day functioning. Short-lived and self-limiting morbidity will usually not be sufficient, but the morbidity need not be irreversible, provided it is persistent or recurrent. Whether a disease or condition is serious is a matter of clinical judgment, based on its impact on such factors as survival, day-to-day functioning, or the likelihood that the disease, if left untreated, will progress from a less severe condition to a more serious one (21 CFR 312.300(b)).

[8] *Federal Register* of August 13, 2009 (74 FR 40900).

[9] For information on the types of regulatory submissions that can be used to obtain expanded access, including treatment IND or treatment protocol, see Q8 in this guidance.

appropriate, of investigational new drugs for treatment use while protecting patient safety and avoiding interference with the development of investigational drugs for marketing under approved applications.

The regulations describe criteria that must be met to authorize expanded access use, requirements for expanded access submissions, and safeguards that are intended to protect patients and preserve the ability to develop meaningful data about the safety and effectiveness of the drug through clinical trials or drug development.

III.　QUESTIONS AND ANSWERS

A.　Expanded Access for Treatment Use

Q1:　What is expanded access?

A1: The terms expanded access, access, and treatment use are used interchangeably to refer to use of an investigational drug when the primary purpose is to diagnose, monitor, or treat a patient's disease or condition. The terms *compassionate use* and *preapproval access* are also occasionally used in the context of the use of an investigational drug to treat a patient. Although these terms have been used informally in the United States and are used outside the United States, they are not defined or described in FDA regulations. This has led to some confusion or lack of clarity about the meaning of the terms (e.g., whether they refer to all expanded access or a type of expanded access, such as individual patient expanded access). For this reason, the terms *compassionate use* and *preapproval access* will not be used in this document.

The main distinction between expanded access and the use of an investigational drug in the usual studies covered under an IND is that expanded access uses are not primarily intended to obtain information about the safety or effectiveness of a drug. Expanded access to an investigational drug can only be provided under a treatment IND or protocol (see Q8) if the sponsor is actively pursuing, with due diligence, marketing approval of the drug for the expanded access use.

Expanded access, access, and treatment use may also refer to (1) use in situations when a drug has been withdrawn for safety reasons, but there exists a patient population for whom the benefits of the withdrawn drug continue to outweigh the risks; (2) use of a similar, but unapproved drug (e.g., foreign-approved drug product) to provide treatment during a drug shortage of the approved drug; (3) use of an approved drug where availability is limited by a risk evaluation and mitigation strategy (REMS) for diagnostic, monitoring, or treatment purposes, by patients who cannot obtain the drug under the REMS; or (4) use for other reasons.

B.   Expanded Access Submissions

Q2:   What types of regulatory submissions can be used to obtain expanded access to a drug under the three expanded access categories?

A2: For each category of expanded access, there are two types of regulatory submissions that can be made: (1) an expanded access protocol submitted as a protocol amendment to an existing IND (i.e., an expanded access protocol) or (2) a new IND submission, which is separate and distinct from any existing INDs and is intended only to make a drug available for treatment use (i.e., an expanded access IND).

A sponsor or physician may contact the appropriate FDA review division for consultation about which may be the most appropriate submission. Additional information about expanded access, including contact information for review divisions, may be found on FDA's Web site at http://www.fda.gov/NewsEvents/PublicHealthFocus/ExpandedAccessCompassionateUse/ucm429610.htm.

Q3:   When should an expanded access protocol submission be used?

A3: An expanded access protocol submission for expanded access should be used only if the sponsor seeking expanded access has an existing IND in effect — typically, such a sponsor is a commercial sponsor with an existing IND under which the sponsor is developing the drug for marketing. When there is an existing IND in effect, FDA generally encourages the submission of an expanded access protocol, rather than a new expanded access IND, because having all expanded access use and clinical trial use consolidated under a single IND may facilitate identification of safety concerns, may make the administrative process less burdensome for sponsors and FDA, and may help in product review.

Q4:   When should a new expanded access IND submission be used?

A4: A new expanded access IND submission for expanded access generally should be used when (1) there is no existing IND in effect for the drug or, more commonly, (2) there is an existing IND in effect for the drug, but the sponsor of the existing IND[10] declines to be the sponsor of the expanded access use (e.g., for an individual patient use, the sponsor of the existing IND may prefer that a patient's physician take on the role of sponsor-investigator and submit a separate individual patient IND).

Q5:   What information should be included in an expanded access submission?

A5: An expanded access submission must include all information required by 21 CFR 312.305(b) and any additional information required for the particular category of expanded access (described in § 312.310(b) for individual patient submissions, in § 312.315(c) for

---

[10] The sponsor of an existing IND typically is the pharmaceutical company or manufacturer of the drug.

intermediate-size patient population submissions, and in § 312.320(b) for treatment submissions), either within the submission itself or by reference to an existing IND.

In cases where the sponsor of an existing IND for the drug has declined to be the sponsor of the expanded access use, the sponsor of that existing IND may give the sponsor of the expanded access IND permission to reference content in the existing IND to satisfy certain requirements for an expanded access IND submission. If permission is obtained, the expanded access IND sponsor should then provide to FDA a letter of authorization (LOA) from the existing IND sponsor (e.g., commercial sponsor/drug manufacturer) that permits FDA to reference that IND.

FDA expects that reference to an existing IND will typically be used by an expanded access IND sponsor to satisfy the requirements to submit the information described in § 312.305(b)(2)(v) (description of the manufacturing facility); in § 312.305(b)(2)(vi) (chemistry, manufacturing, and controls information); and in § 312.305(b)(2)(vii) (pharmacology and toxicology information).

IND submissions that reference an existing IND generally will include the information described in §§ 312.305(b)(2)(ii), (iii), (iv), and (viii) and in § 312.305(b)(3) in the expanded access IND submission. As noted, the expanded access submission must also include the additional information that may be required for the specific category of expanded access.

See Q9 for information on the forms that are available to use for expanded access submissions.

Q6: Is institutional review board (IRB) review and approval required for all expanded access categories?

A6: Except for emergency expanded access use (see Q8) when there is not sufficient time to secure prospective IRB review, an investigator treating a patient with an investigational drug under expanded access is responsible for obtaining IRB review[11] and approval consistent with 21 CFR part 56 before treatment with the investigational drug may begin, regardless of whether the protocol is submitted in a new IND or to an existing IND (21 CFR 312.305(c)(4)). In the case of emergency expanded access use, FDA authorization is still required (§ 312.310(d)), but it is not necessary to wait for IRB approval to begin treatment. However, the IRB must be notified of the emergency expanded access use within 5 working days of emergency use (§ 56.104(c)).

---

[11] An institutional review board (IRB) means any board, committee, or other group formally designated by an institution to review, to approve the initiation of, and to conduct periodic review of biomedical research involving human subjects. The primary purpose of IRB review is to assure that the rights and welfare of human subjects are protected, including by determining that informed consent is obtained in accordance with and to the extent required by Federal requirements. Many institutions have their own IRB to oversee human subjects research conducted within the institution or by the staff of the institution. If the patient's physician does not have access to a local IRB, an independent IRB may be used. The Department of Health and Human Services' Office for Human Research Protections maintains a database of registered IRBs. Go to http://ohrp.cit.nih.gov/search/irbsearch.aspx?styp=bsc and click on "Advanced Search." Enter your state to find registered IRBs in your area. For more information see http://www.fda.gov/NewsEvents/PublicHealthFocus/ExpandedAccessCompassionateUse/default.htm.

Part 56 requires, among other things, that the IRB review the expanded access use at a convened meeting at which a majority of the IRB members are present (*full IRB review*) (§ 56.108(c)).

FDA is aware of concerns that this requirement for full IRB review may deter individual patient expanded access to investigational drugs for treatment use. The concerns are primarily about IRB review of individual patient expanded access INDs and protocols in settings in which IRB review is not readily accessible (e.g., health care settings that do not have IRBs). Although patients seeking expanded access may be in dire clinical circumstances under which ethical oversight is particularly important, we do not want to deter expanded access for individual patients. We have encouraged use of central IRBs for review of expanded access uses. However, other options may be needed, and FDA will consider proposed options that might better facilitate individual patient expanded access while providing appropriate ethical oversight.

Q7: Are expanded access submissions subject to the informed consent requirements?

A7: Yes. Expanded access to an investigational drug for treatment use, including emergency use, requires informed consent as described in 21 CFR part 50, unless one of the exceptions found in part 50 applies.[12] Investigators treating a patient(s) with an investigational drug under expanded access are responsible for ensuring that the informed consent requirements of part 50 are met (21 CFR 312.305(c)(4)). One of the purposes of informed consent is to ensure that the patient is informed that he/she will be treated with an investigational product and that there may be uncertainty about the safety and effectiveness of the product. The provision in § 50.25(a)(1) specifies that the consent include "a statement that the study involves research, an explanation of the purposes of the research and the expected duration of the subject's participation, a description of the procedures to be followed, and identification of any procedures which are experimental."

Q8: How does FDA categorize and subcategorize expanded access submissions?

A8: FDA distinguishes among expanded access INDs and expanded access protocols, the three different categories of expanded access and, for individual patient expanded access, between emergency and non-emergency individual patient expanded access.

This results in the following sub-categorization of expanded access submissions:

Individual Patient Expanded Access, Including for Emergency Use
    1) Individual patient expanded access IND
        1a) Individual patient expanded access IND for emergency use

---

[12] For information on informed consent in general, see the draft guidance for industry *Informed Consent Information Sheet – Guidance for IRBs, Clinical Investigators, and Sponsors*. When final, this guidance will represent FDA's current thinking on this topic. For additional information on the part 50 informed consent exceptions, see the guidance for institutional review boards, clinical investigators, and sponsors *Exception from Informed Consent Requirements for Emergency Research*.

2) Individual patient expanded access protocol
      2a) Individual patient expanded access protocol for emergency use

<u>Intermediate-Size Patient Populations</u>
     1) Intermediate-size patient population expanded access IND
     2) Intermediate-size patient population expanded access protocol

<u>Treatment IND or Treatment Protocol (expanded access for widespread use)</u>
     1) Treatment IND
     2) Treatment protocol

Individual Patient Expanded Access, Including for Emergency Use (also referred to as single patient expanded access)

1) **Individual patient expanded access IND** (also referred to as single patient IND): Expanded access to an investigational drug for treatment use by a single patient submitted under a new IND. Unless FDA notifies the sponsor (e.g., the patient's physician) that treatment may begin earlier, there is a 30-day period from the date FDA receives the IND before treatment with the drug may begin (21 CFR 312.305(d)(1)).

    1a) Individual patient expanded access IND for emergency use: A subset of individual patient INDs that provide expanded access to an investigational drug for treatment use by a single patient in an emergency situation (i.e., a situation that requires a patient to be treated before a written submission can be made) submitted under a new IND (21 CFR 312.310(d)). Treatment is initially requested and authorized by telephone (or other rapid means of communication) and may start immediately upon FDA authorization, and the physician or sponsor must agree to submit a written submission (IND) within 15 working days of the initial authorization (§ 312.310(d)(2)).

2) **Individual patient expanded access protocol** (also referred to as single patient protocol): Expanded access to an investigational drug for treatment use by a single patient submitted as a protocol to an existing IND by the sponsor of the existing IND. There is no 30-day period before treatment with the drug may begin, but the protocol must be submitted to FDA and have IRB approval consistent with 21 CFR part 56 (see 21 CFR 312.305(c)(4)) before treatment may begin. (See §§ 312.305(d)(2) and 312.30(a).)

    2a) Individual patient expanded access protocol for emergency use: An emergency use protocol is a subset of individual patient protocols that provides expanded access to an investigational drug for treatment use by a single patient in an emergency situation (i.e., a situation that requires a patient to be treated before a written submission can be made) submitted as a protocol to an existing IND by the sponsor of the existing IND (21 CFR 312.310(d)). Treatment is initially requested and authorized by telephone (or other rapid means of communication) and may start immediately upon FDA authorization, with a requirement for a written submission (protocol) to FDA within 15 working days of the initial authorization (§ 312.310(d)(2)).

In an emergency situation (either an emergency use IND or emergency use protocol) when there is not sufficient time to secure IRB review prior to beginning treatment, the emergency use of the investigational drug must be reported to the IRB within 5 working days of emergency use, as required under § 56.104(c).

Contact information for emergency use INDs and protocols is located on FDA's expanded access Web site at http://www.fda.gov/NewsEvents/PublicHealthFocus/ExpandedAccessCompassionate Use/default.htm.

Intermediate-Size Patient Population Expanded Access

1) **Intermediate-size patient population expanded access IND**: Expanded access to an investigational drug for use by more than one patient, but generally fewer patients than are treated under a typical treatment IND or protocol, submitted under a new IND. Unless FDA notifies the sponsor that treatment may begin earlier, there is a 30-day period from the date FDA receives the IND before treatment with the drug may begin (21 CFR 312.305(d)(1)).

2) **Intermediate-size patient population expanded access protocol**: Expanded access to an investigational drug for use by more than one patient, but generally fewer patients than are treated under a typical treatment IND or protocol, submitted as a protocol to an existing IND by the sponsor of the existing IND. There is no 30-day period before treatment with the drug may begin, but the protocol must be submitted to FDA and have IRB approval before treatment with the drug may begin. (See 21 CFR 312.305(d)(2) and 312.30(a).)

For more information about intermediate-size patient population expanded access, see Q18 and Q19.

Treatment IND or Treatment Protocol

1) **Treatment IND**: Expanded access to an investigational drug for treatment use by a large (widespread) population, submitted under a new IND. Unless FDA notifies the sponsor that treatment may begin earlier, there is a 30-day period from the date FDA receives the IND before treatment with the drug may begin (21 CFR 312.305(d)(1)).

2) **Treatment protocol**: Expanded access to an investigational drug for treatment use generally by a large (widespread) population, submitted as a protocol to an existing IND by the sponsor of the existing IND. Unlike other expanded access protocols submitted to existing INDs, there is a 30-day period from the date FDA receives the

protocol before treatment with the drug may begin unless FDA notifies the sponsor that treatment may begin earlier (21 CFR 312.305(d)(2)(ii)).

FDA recommends that the expanded access submission identify the relevant subcategory.

C.   Individual (or Single) Patient Expanded Access

Q9:   What forms are used with individual patient expanded access submissions?

A9: Individual patient INDs, including for emergency use, submitted by a licensed physician (sponsor-investigator), may be submitted using Form FDA 1571 (Investigational New Drug Application (IND)), which is a transmittal form that accompanies the IND and provides information to identify the type of submission and its contents. However, the physician may instead choose to submit the IND using Form FDA 3926 (Individual Patient Expanded Access Investigational New Drug Application (IND)), which, when completed (including attachments, if appropriate), constitutes the individual patient IND submission. Form FDA 3926 is a streamlined alternative and was created specifically for individual patient IND submissions, including those for emergency use.

For individual patient INDs and for individual patient protocols submitted to an existing IND *by a commercial sponsor*, Form FDA 1571 should accompany the submission. The most current version of all FDA forms can be downloaded from the FDA Web site at http://www.fda.gov/AboutFDA/ReportsManualsForms/Forms/default.htm.

For both forms, when the submitter and the physician treating the patient are the same, the patient's physician should be identified as the sponsor. By signing the form, the physician (as sponsor-investigator) agrees to all the items contained in the form, including seeking IRB review and approval and informed consent for the expanded access use.

The following chart illustrates which form may be used for each type of submission:

Table 1. Acceptable Expanded Access Submission Forms		
	Form FDA 3926	Form FDA 1571
Individual patient IND submitted by a licensed physician	✓	✓
Individual patient protocol		✓
Individual patient IND for emergency use submitted by a licensed physician	✓	✓
Individual patient protocol for emergency use		✓
Intermediate-size patient population IND		✓
Intermediate-size patient population protocol		✓
Treatment IND		✓
Treatment protocol		✓

Q10: Who can make a submission for individual patient expanded access?

A10: The sponsor of an existing IND under which a drug is being developed (e.g., a pharmaceutical company or manufacturer of the investigational drug) or a licensed physician may make an individual patient expanded access submission (21 CFR 312.310(b)(1)).

The sponsor of an existing IND (e.g., a pharmaceutical company or manufacturer of the investigational drug) can submit an individual patient expanded access protocol to its existing IND. In this scenario, the sponsor of the existing IND is also the sponsor of the expanded access protocol, and the patient's physician is the investigator for the expanded access protocol. The term *investigator* is used because the drug is investigational, but does not denote the physician's or patient's involvement in clinical research.

The sponsor of the existing IND can instead submit an individual patient expanded access IND and cross-reference information in its existing IND to support the individual patient expanded access IND. In this scenario, the sponsor of the existing IND is also the sponsor of the expanded access IND, and the patient's physician is the investigator for the expanded access IND.

Because having all clinical trials and expanded access use requests for a drug under a single IND may facilitate identification of safety concerns, ease the administrative burden for both sponsors and FDA, and will help in product review (if the drug is under development for marketing), it is preferable for sponsors to submit an individual patient expanded access protocol to an existing IND when possible.

A physician can submit an individual patient expanded access IND for his/her patient. In this scenario, when the patient's physician submits an expanded access IND, the physician is both the sponsor and the investigator—in other words, he or she is considered a sponsor-investigator (§ 312.305(c)(3)) for the purposes of part 312. The physician may satisfy some of the expanded access submission requirements by referring to information in an existing IND if the physician obtains permission from the sponsor of the existing IND (see Q5). If the physician obtains this permission from the sponsor of the existing IND, the physician should provide to FDA the LOA from the sponsor of the IND that permits FDA to reference the sponsor's IND.

In cases where it is not possible to obtain an LOA (e.g., the entity supplying the drug does not have an IND filed with FDA), physicians should contact the relevant FDA review division to determine what information is needed to support the expanded access submission. Physicians should also contact the review division if the individual patient expanded access IND is for an approved drug where availability is limited by a REMS. The physician should then submit an individual patient expanded access IND to the appropriate FDA review division and may choose to use Form FDA 3926.[13] Contact information for review divisions may be found on FDA's Web site at http://www.fda.gov/NewsEvents/PublicHealthFocus/ExpandedAccessCompassionateUse/ucm42 9610.htm. If the sponsor of the existing IND (e.g., commercial sponsor or drug manufacturer) does not authorize reference to the IND, the physician sponsoring the expanded access IND must include in the IND all the information required to support the expanded access IND (§ 312.310).

A patient's physician may not submit an individual patient expanded access protocol to an existing IND for which the physician is not the sponsor.

Regardless of who is the sponsor of an individual patient expanded access protocol or expanded access IND, the patient can obtain expanded access to the investigational drug only through treatment by a licensed physician (§ 312.310).

Q11: What are the roles of the patient's physician and FDA in determining if expanded access for an individual patient is appropriate?

A11: FDA may permit expanded access to a drug for an individual patient when the criteria in 21 CFR 312.305(a), applicable to all types of expanded access, and the criteria in § 312.310(a), specific to individual patient expanded access, are met. For these criteria to be met, both the patient's physician and FDA must make certain determinations.

The patient's physician must determine that the probable risk to the patient from the investigational drug is not greater than the probable risk from the disease or condition (§ 312.310(a)(1)). The physician should make this determination based on the information about the drug available to the physician and the physician's knowledge of the patient's clinical situation.

As with all types of expanded access, FDA must determine, based on the information available to FDA, that the potential benefit justifies the potential risks of the treatment use with the drug and that those risks are not unreasonable in the context of the disease or condition to be treated

---

[13] Form FDA 3926 and accompanying instructions may be found on FDA's Web site at http://www.fda.gov/AboutFDA/ReportsManualsForms/Forms/default.htm.

(§ 312.305(a)(2)). To authorize the expanded access use, FDA must also determine (1) that the patient has a serious or life-threatening disease or condition and has no other comparable or satisfactory therapeutic options (§ 312.305(a)(1)); (2) that providing expanded access will not interfere with development of the drug for the expanded access use (§ 312.305(a)(3)); and (3) that the patient cannot obtain the drug under another IND or protocol (§ 312.310(a)(2)) (e.g., in a clinical study of the drug).

Q12: What are some of the reasons for FDA to deny a request for individual patient expanded access when previous requests for the same drug for the same or a similar use have been permitted?

A12: Each request for individual patient expanded access to a drug should be treated as a unique clinical situation, and the risks and benefits should be evaluated based on that clinical situation. Even when there are two (or more) individual patient expanded access requests for patients with the same disease or condition, there may be significant differences in the clinical presentation of the disease or condition that make the risks acceptable for one patient, but not for another. For example, a patient may have a different stage of the disease or different tumor type than previous patients who were permitted expanded access to the drug and, therefore, may have a different benefit/risk ratio. Similarly, a patient may have a comorbid condition not present in previous patients who obtained expanded access that would make the risk unacceptable. FDA may also become aware of new safety signals or information about effectiveness that changes the benefit/risk ratio such that the risk is no longer acceptable for the patient. In cases such as these, individual patient expanded access for additional patients might be denied.

There also may be nonclinical reasons for denying expanded access. For example, a patient seeking expanded access may be able to enroll in a clinical trial that was not accessible to a previous patient who was granted expanded access (e.g., because the previous patient met criteria for exclusion from the trial or the trial was geographically inaccessible to the previous patient). FDA could also have become aware since authorizing previous requests for expanded access that expanded access is impeding the clinical development of the drug and, on that basis, deny further requests for expanded access.

Q13: How does FDA address individual patient expanded access applications for treatment with multiple courses of therapy or treatment of a chronic condition?

A13: Under 21 CFR 312.310(c)(1), individual patient expanded access is generally limited to a single course of therapy for a specified duration. However, as reflected in § 312.310(c)(1), FDA may authorize multiple courses of therapy or chronic therapy for individual patient expanded access, including authorizing individual patient expanded access to treat a chronic disease or condition that requires extended treatment. FDA generally authorizes such individual patient expanded access when the circumstances of the treatment are well defined and reasonable in light of the available evidence to support use of the drug. The patient's physician (as the investigator) proposes the full course of treatment when filing the request for expanded access. To fairly weigh the risks and benefits of a drug for use for individual patient expanded access, FDA believes the planned course of therapy should be well defined because it will usually be necessary to consider the planned dose and duration of therapy in relation to what is known about the occurrence of toxicity for that dose and duration of therapy. Therefore, FDA typically authorizes expanded access for an extended duration for the treatment of a chronic condition when the patient's condition and the information available about the safety of the drug support an extended duration of treatment, but FDA does not typically authorize expanded access for an unspecified duration at the discretion of the patient's physician. For example, FDA may authorize expanded access of extended duration for a drug being developed to treat multiple sclerosis or other types of progressively debilitating neuromuscular disease if it is critical that the drug be administered chronically to slow the progression of the disease and if the information available about the safety of the drug supports an extended duration of treatment. If expanded access use is authorized for an extended duration, FDA may require the sponsor to continue to monitor the individual patient expanded access use through the extended duration (see § 312.310(c)(3)).

Q14: When should individual patient expanded access using the emergency procedures in 21 CFR 312.310(d) be requested?

A14: Section 312.310(d) states that FDA may authorize expanded access for an individual patient without a written submission if there is "an emergency that requires the patient to be treated before a written submission can be made." The licensed physician or sponsor, however, must agree to submit an expanded access IND or protocol within 15 working days of FDA's authorization of the use (§ 312.310(d)(2)). FDA believes this regulation means that it is appropriate to request individual patient expanded access using the emergency procedures described in § 312.310(d) when treatment of the patient must occur within a very limited number of hours or days. FDA intends to authorize expanded access for such requests only when the situation is a true emergency.

Q15: Can the same drug be used in an emergency situation at the same institution more than once? If so, is prospective IRB review required for the subsequent expanded access emergency use?

A15: There can be more than one expanded access emergency use of the same drug at the same institution. For expanded access uses authorized under the emergency procedures, the emergency use must be reported to the responsible IRB within 5 working days of initiation of treatment (21 CFR 56.104(c)). Generally, once an investigational drug is used in an emergency situation without prior IRB approval, any subsequent uses of the investigational drug at that same institution would require prior IRB review and approval (§ 56.104(c)). An institution or physician that expects subsequent use of the investigational drug should request review and approval by the appropriate IRB after the initial emergency use. However, when prior IRB review and approval is not feasible for a subsequent expanded access emergency use at a particular institution, FDA does not intend to deny the subsequent request for emergency use based on lack of time to obtain prospective IRB review, as long as that use will be reported to the IRB within 5 working days of initiation of treatment (§ 56.104(c)).

Q16: Can a commercial sponsor provide emergency expanded access to its investigational drug to multiple patients?

A16: While most emergency individual patient expanded access is obtained through individual patient expanded access INDs for emergency use, a commercial sponsor (i.e., the pharmaceutical company or drug manufacturer that is developing the drug for marketing) can provide emergency expanded access to its investigational drug to an individual patient who requires treatment before a written submission can be made through an emergency use protocol to the commercial sponsor's existing commercial IND. A separate request would be needed for each patient seeking expanded access, but the commercial sponsor can make multiple such requests under its existing IND.

In such cases, the IND sponsor is the commercial sponsor and must agree to submit an expanded access protocol for each separate request to its existing IND within 15 working days of FDA's authorization of the use (21 CFR 312.310(d)(2)). Furthermore, although this emergency use is exempt from prior IRB review, as described 21 CFR 56.104(c), the emergency use must be reported to the appropriate IRB within 5 working days of emergency use.

D.   Intermediate-Size Patient Population and Treatment INDs and Protocols

Q17: Can there be more than one intermediate-size patient population expanded access IND or protocol for a particular drug for the same disease or condition?

A17: When multiple patients with the same disease or condition seek expanded access to a particular drug and the relevant criteria for expanded access are met, FDA believes that it is generally most efficient to consolidate expanded access in a single intermediate-size patient population IND or protocol. If the drug is being developed, FDA believes it is most efficient if the commercial sponsor is the sponsor of a single intermediate-size patient population expanded access IND or protocol. However, the regulations do not preclude the possibility of authorizing more than one intermediate-size patient population expanded access IND or protocol, with different sponsors or sponsor-investigators, for a drug for the same disease or condition. Thus, there may be situations in which there are multiple intermediate-size patient population expanded access INDs or protocols for a drug for the treatment of the same disease or condition. FDA expects these situations to arise infrequently.

Q18: When is it appropriate to request expanded access for multiple patients using an intermediate-size patient population expanded access IND or protocol rather than a treatment IND or protocol?

A18: FDA regulations do not impose specific numerical limitations for when an intermediate-size patient population expanded access IND or protocol (as opposed to a treatment IND or protocol) may be appropriate. This determination generally depends on the following two factors:

1. *Whether the drug is under development for marketing for the expanded access use*

If the drug is not being developed for marketing and the expanded access IND or protocol is intended to treat more than a single patient, expanded access would be provided under an intermediate-size patient population expanded access. Expanded access to an investigational drug can only be provided under a treatment IND or protocol if the drug is being developed for marketing for the expanded access use. When the investigational drug is being developed, intermediate-size patient population expanded access is used earlier in development than treatment INDs or protocols. Also, if clinical development of the drug is essentially complete (i.e., the clinical trials to support marketing approval of the investigational drug have ended) and the intent of the expanded access is to bridge the gap (to ensure that treatment is not interrupted and to expand treatment to additional patients) between completion of the clinical trials and marketing of the drug, the expanded access, regardless of the number of patients expected to be treated, would generally be designated as a treatment IND or protocol.

2. *Size of the patient population*

The second factor important to a determination of whether expanded access is provided under an intermediate-size patient population expanded access (as opposed to a treatment IND or protocol) is the size of the patient population. In general, intermediate-size patient population expanded access is intended to accommodate population sizes smaller than the large populations typical of treatment INDs or protocols. However, as noted in the preceding paragraph, if clinical development is complete and the intent of the expanded access IND or protocol is to bridge the gap between the completion of clinical trials and marketing, expanded access would generally be provided under a treatment IND or protocol, regardless of the intended size of the patient population. Similarly, if the drug is not being developed for marketing for the expanded access use, expanded access would be provided under an intermediate-size patient population IND or protocol, regardless of the size of the patient population (as long as it is intended to treat more than a single patient).

Separate single patient INDs may be combined into a single intermediate-size patient population protocol when feasible and practical, at the request of the sponsor or the FDA. Adding patients to an intermediate-size patient population protocol can reduce paperwork and simplify IRB review. In such cases, any number beyond one patient might be reasonable. When a growing number of eligible patients might benefit from treatment access under an intermediate-size patient population protocol, a treatment IND may be appropriate. (See Q19.)

Q19: **The regulations in 21 CFR 312.315(d)(iii) state that as enrollment in an intermediate-size patient population expanded access IND or protocol increases, FDA may ask the sponsor to submit an IND or protocol for the use under 312.320 (i.e., to transition the intermediate-size patient population expanded access IND or protocol to a treatment expanded access IND or protocol). When and how would FDA make such a determination and how would such a transition be carried out?**

A19: FDA anticipates that there would ordinarily be a seamless transition from intermediate-size patient population expanded access to expanded access under a treatment IND or protocol at the point when the evidence is sufficient to support the treatment IND or protocol, when there is adequate progress with drug development, and when the sponsor is willing to make the drug available to a potentially larger patient population under a treatment IND or protocol. Although there will be a 30-day period for initiation of the new treatment IND or protocol, as required by the regulations, the review division can act sooner and FDA may notify the sponsor that treatment may begin earlier (21 CFR 312.40 and 312.305(d)(1)).

For such a transition, all patients currently receiving treatment with the investigational drug would continue treatment under the intermediate-size patient population expanded access IND or protocol until they transition to the treatment IND or protocol (to ensure that treatment is not interrupted). Once all patients in the intermediate-size patient population expanded access IND or protocol are receiving their treatment under the new treatment IND or protocol, the intermediate-size patient population expanded access IND or protocol will be terminated.

E.   Time Frame for Beginning Treatment Under an Expanded Access IND or Protocol

Q20:   When can access for emergency use begin?

A20: For an emergency use, expanded access to the drug may begin upon authorization (usually provided by telephone or other rapid means of communication) by the reviewing FDA official (21 CFR 312.305(d)(2)(i), with a requirement for a written submission (protocol) to FDA within 15 working days of the initial authorization (§ 312.310(d)(2)). As explained in Q15, FDA expects that for expanded access uses authorized under the emergency procedures, there typically will not be time to obtain prior IRB approval of the use. In such cases, the emergency use must be reported to the responsible IRB within 5 working days of initiation of treatment (21 CFR 56.104(c)).

Q21:   When can treatment begin under expanded access INDs not for emergency use?

A21: When an expanded access IND (not for emergency use) is submitted, the treatment use of the drug may begin when the IND goes into effect and IRB approval has been obtained consistent with 21 CFR part 56 (see 21 CFR 312.305(c)(4)). As is true for any new IND, an expanded access IND goes into effect 30 days after FDA receives the IND (unless the IND is put on clinical hold, i.e., is not allowed to proceed) or on earlier notification by FDA (§§ 312.40 and 312.305(d)(1)).

Q22:   When can treatment begin under expanded access protocols not for emergency use?

A22: For an individual patient or intermediate-size patient population expanded access protocol, expanded access to the drug can begin once the expanded access protocol has been submitted to FDA and has been approved by an IRB (21 CFR 312.305(d)(2)). For a treatment protocol, however, expanded access may not begin until 30 days after FDA receives the protocol (or on earlier notification by FDA (§ 312.305(d)(2)(ii)) and IRB approval has been obtained consistent with 21 CFR part 56 (see 21 CFR 312.305(c)(4)).

F.   General Questions

Q23:   Can FDA require a company to provide expanded access to its drug if FDA authorizes the expanded access?

A23: No. FDA cannot compel a company to provide expanded access to its drug. When a company provides expanded access to its drug, it does so voluntarily.

Q24:   How does FDA determine that authorizing expanded access to a drug will not interfere with clinical trials or drug development?

A24: Under 21 CFR 312.305(a)(3), to authorize any category of expanded access, FDA must determine that expanded access to the drug for the requested use will not interfere with the initiation, conduct, or completion of clinical investigations that could support marketing approval of the expanded access use or otherwise compromise the potential development of the drug for the expanded access use. Generally, patients must be ineligible or otherwise unable (e.g., geographically unable to access a study site) to enter ongoing clinical trials to receive the drug under an expanded access IND or protocol. For all categories of expanded access, sponsors are required to include in their access submissions information adequate to demonstrate that expanded access to the drug will not interfere with clinical investigations or drug development, along with other information (§§ 312.310(b), 312.315(c), and 312.320(b)).

FDA believes that expanded access INDs or protocols that treat larger patient populations generally have the greatest potential to interfere with clinical investigations or drug development, because of their greater potential to interfere with recruiting patients for the clinical investigation(s). FDA typically determines whether an expanded access use will interfere with clinical investigations or drug development based on the information provided by the sponsor in its expanded access submission. If the information provided by the sponsor is not adequate for FDA to make this determination, FDA may ask the sponsor for additional information.

For example, before authorizing a treatment IND for a drug for which clinical trials are ongoing, FDA may ask the sponsor to explain how the sponsor will ensure that the treatment IND will not interfere with accrual of patients in the clinical trials, and how the sponsor will determine whether interference is occurring, if such information is not provided in the expanded access submission. More specifically, FDA may ask the sponsor to submit to its IND a comprehensive investigational plan with a timetable and milestones (if it has not done so already) so that FDA can periodically assess whether the treatment IND is affecting accrual of patients in the clinical trials or other parameters related to the pace of drug development. If FDA then determines that the ongoing treatment IND is interfering with clinical trials or drug development or that the sponsor is not pursuing, with due diligence, marketing approval for the expanded access use, FDA could place the treatment IND on clinical hold (§ 312.42(b)(3)).

Q25: What data and information must sponsors submit as follow-up for approved expanded access INDs or protocols?

A25: As with any IND, in all cases of expanded access, sponsors are responsible for submitting IND safety reports and annual reports (when the IND or protocol continues for 1 year or longer) to FDA as required under 21 CFR 312.32 and 312.33 (see § 312.305(c)).

For individual patient expanded access, the regulations in § 312.310(c)(2) specify that, at the conclusion of treatment, the sponsor must provide to FDA a written summary of the results of the expanded access use, including adverse effects.

From a public health perspective, early identification of important adverse events is beneficial. For example, a relatively rare adverse event might be detected during expanded access use, or such use might contribute safety information for a population not exposed to the drug in clinical trials. There are a small number of cases in which FDA has used adverse event information from expanded access in the safety assessment of a drug. However, FDA reviewers of these adverse event data understand the context in which the expanded access use was permitted (e.g., use in patients with serious or immediately life-threatening diseases or administered in a clinical setting (not clinical trial) and will evaluate any adverse event data obtained from an expanded access submission within that context.

Expanded access INDs and protocols are generally not designed to determine the efficacy of a drug; however, the expanded access regulations do not prohibit the collection of such data. Because expanded access INDs or protocols typically involve uncontrolled exposures (with limited data collection), it is unlikely that an expanded access IND or protocol would yield efficacy information that would be useful to FDA in considering a drug's effectiveness.

Q26: Can FDA consider an IND or protocol submission to be an expanded access submission and identify and review it as such, even though the applicant does not identify it as an expanded access submission?

A26: Yes. For example, FDA intends to evaluate whether proposals for studies described as open-label safety studies should be considered treatment INDs or protocols. The goal of an open-label safety study is to better characterize the safety of a drug late in its development. However, in practice, many studies that are described as open-label safety studies have characteristics that appear to be more consistent with treatment INDs or protocols. If an IND or protocol describes an open-label study that provides for broad expanded access to an investigational drug in the later stages of development, but lacks planned, systematic data collection and a design adequate to meaningfully evaluate a safety issue, FDA will generally consider the submission to be a treatment IND or protocol. In the event that a protocol is not submitted as an expanded access protocol, but is designated as such by FDA, the review division will notify the sponsor of the designation.

Q27: **What is the difference between an expanded access protocol and a continuation or open-label safety protocol?**

A27: A continuation protocol describes a trial in which patients are allowed to remain on an investigational drug or cross over to an investigational drug from placebo or active control following conclusion of the randomized phase of a trial. An open-label safety study is an uncontrolled trial (i.e., there is no comparison or control group). The primary purpose of both continuation and open-label safety protocols, in contrast to expanded access protocols, is to obtain safety data on the investigational drug. The conduct of continuation and open-label safety protocols differs from that of expanded access protocols in that (1) participation in open-label safety and continuation protocols is usually limited to specific, named institutions/centers; (2) participating investigators in continuation or open-label safety protocols are already identified and trained to collect needed safety data; and (3) in the case of a continuation trial, participants are typically limited to those in the original randomized, controlled trial.

Q28: **If a sponsor continues to provide its investigational drug for treatment use under its IND to a patient who was enrolled in a clinical trial, but who does not continue to meet inclusion criteria, is that considered expanded access (i.e., is the sponsor expected to make an expanded access submission to continue to provide the drug to that patient)?**

A28: In general, if a patient is already enrolled in a clinical trial (designed to further the development of or determine the safety and/or effectiveness of an investigational drug) and the patient's results are to be included in the analysis of the investigational drug, the continued treatment of that patient with the investigational drug is not considered expanded access, even if the patient does not continue to meet all the study inclusion criteria or the patient's treatment deviates from the study protocol. This is commonly known as a protocol exception and would be covered under the existing IND.

Q29: **If a sponsor provides its investigational drug for treatment use under its IND to a patient who does not meet inclusion criteria for their trial and is not enrolled in the trial, is that considered expanded access?**

A29: In general, if a patient is not enrolled in a clinical trial but is provided expanded access to the investigational drug for the purposes of treating the patient, treatment of that patient with the investigational drug is considered expanded access to the investigational drug, and the sponsor should meet the requirements for expanded access.

Q30: **How can patients and health care providers determine if a company is providing or is willing to provide expanded access to an investigational drug?**

A30: Information on publicly and privately supported clinical trials on a wide range of diseases and conditions is available at ClinicalTrials.gov, a Web-based resource maintained by the National Library of Medicine for patients, their families, health care professionals, researchers, and the public.

When registering its trial at ClinicalTrials.gov, the individual or entity registering the trial is asked whether expanded access is available for the investigational drug and, if so, is prompted to provide certain information about obtaining such expanded access. This information on expanded access is then included on the ClinicalTrials.gov Web site.

Not all clinical trials must be registered on ClinicalTrials.gov, and in most cases expanded access trials are not required to be registered (although they may be registered voluntarily). Therefore the fact that an expanded access trial is not registered on ClinicalTrials.gov may not mean that expanded access is not available for a particular investigational drug outside of the clinical trial(s). Physicians or patients may inquire with the sponsor (or manufacturer of the investigational drug, if different from the sponsor) about possible availability. Because expanded access to an investigational drug is provided under an IND and information within and pertaining to an IND is generally not publicly available, the best source other than ClinicalTrials.gov for information on expanded access to a particular investigational drug, such as whether expanded access is available or who to contact to obtain expanded access, is the sponsor of the IND or the manufacturer of the investigational drug. Sometimes the sponsor or manufacturer will include such information on their Web site. FDA encourages companies that are developing drugs for the treatment of serious diseases, especially those for which the clinical development program has been granted fast-track or breakthrough therapy designation, to make contact information and information about their company's expanded access programs and policies available to the public.

Q31: May treatment with two or more investigational drugs be requested and authorized under a single expanded access IND or protocol or may an individual patient participate in more than one expanded access IND or protocol (e.g., be enrolled in two different treatment INDs)?

A31: Yes. A single expanded access IND or protocol may involve treatment with more than one investigational drug, and a patient may be enrolled in more than one expanded access IND or protocol. When expanded access to two or more investigational drugs is needed to treat a single disease and the relevant criteria are met, it is most efficient to provide expanded access to the multiple investigational drugs under a single expanded access IND or protocol, rather than to provide expanded access by having a patient enroll in two or more separate expanded access INDs or protocols (one for each drug). Management of the patient's disease, treatment, and the collection of information about the therapy is likely to be better coordinated under a single expanded access IND or protocol.